GOING FOR IT
Becoming the Healthiest You

Brian Narelle & Robert W. Adams, DC, DABCN
Board Certified in Chiropractic Neurology
Forward by Prof. Ted Carrick

Going For It
Becoming The Healthiest You

Limits of Liability/Disclaimer of Warranty

1st Printing January 2018
Printed in the United States of America

To better health from:

Dr. Robert Adams continues his contribution to humankind with his latest installments in his entertaining and informative health trilogy. *Going for It: Becoming the Healthiest You* is another must read. The book is a joy for those people that demand an understanding of themselves. It is concise and simple while embracing the complexity associated with the human brain and nervous system.   Difficult concepts are immediately understandable by the use of cartoons.   This book, the third in a series, promotes autonomy of the individual by presenting us with things that we might be able to do by ourselves and for ourselves. Uniquely, there are no costs involved to undertake the recommendations that Dr. Adams presents. Lifestyle modifications and changes including exercise based upon the knowledge of human systems are central to this contribution. This book stimulates the reader to do things for him/herself with a realistic probability of success. Adams presents five keys to the very best "you" with great news that the keys are already in our pockets. I found this unique in comparison to the multitude of self health literature available. The reader has an understanding of them self and what is necessary to do the best things for their health with easy to do exercises that can be done in the home. We are presented with a choice and it is clear that Dr. Adams wants to prepare us to be the people that are in control of their own health care destiny. His recommendations are contemporary, realistic and rather simple to include in one's lifestyle. This is an easy read and one that will have a consequence for everyone that might be lucky enough to pick it up. It is a superior contribution to humankind and I am very pleased to have read it and to recommend it.

Prof. Frederick R. Carrick, DC, PhD, MS-HPed
Roland Blaauw Professor of Neurology and
Senior Research Fellow BCMHR in association with
University of Cambridge

DEDICATION

Going For It: Becoming the Healthiest You is dedicated to my four wonders: Joshua, Kylee, Zachary and Lucas. They have been tremendous blessing to Jamie and I. We have been inspired and educated by them in essential life lessons. I have grown and gained wisdom from their influence.

Robert W. Adams

MISSION ACCOMPLISHED...ALMOST

While we would have never made it to the moon without a thorough understanding of all the systems involved, understanding without action wouldn't have gotten us very far.

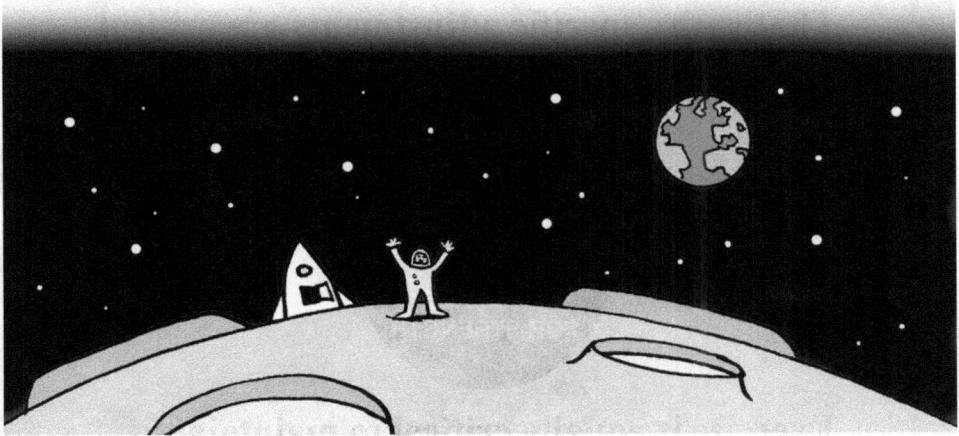

When it comes to your body, understanding the relationship of movement receptors and your brain's regulation of muscle protein is a key to achieving optimal health.

But action is required on your part: including periodic adjustments as well as regular exercise. Remember, muscle protein has a half life of only 6-10 days.

CONSCIOUS CONTROL

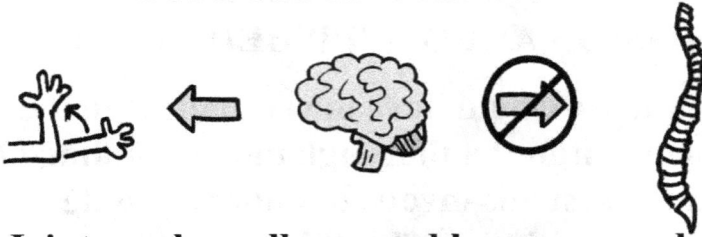

Joints such as elbows and knees are under our conscious control. Spinal joints are not. That's why specific adjustments are critical to restoring full range of motion.

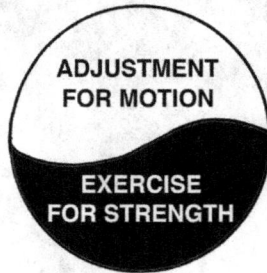

ADJUSTMENT FOR MOTION

EXERCISE FOR STRENGTH

Exercise is equally critical to maintaining postural integrity. Remember, motion is critical to activating movement receptors, which in turn stimulate muscle protein. This combination is your ticket out of the neck and back pain that plagues so many. Pain that often leads to opioid abuse...

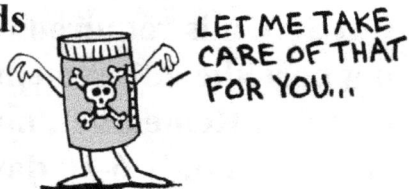

LET ME TAKE CARE OF THAT FOR YOU...

TROUBLE DOWN BELOW

Dulling pain with drugs does nothing to resolve the underlying problems. Low back and leg pain often have their origins higher up.

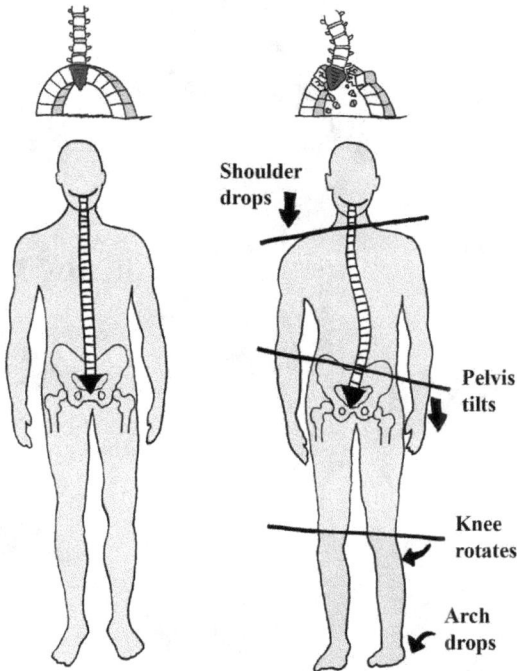

Shoulder drops

Pelvis tilts

Knee rotates

Arch drops

Any imbalance requires compensation... and compensations create their own problems. That's why alignment and strength throughout your body are important.

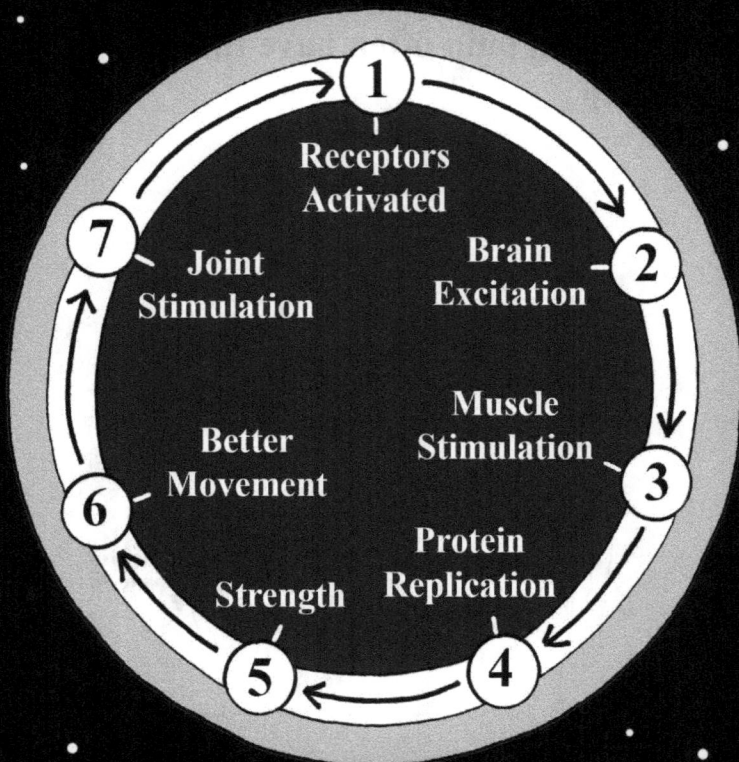

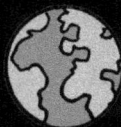

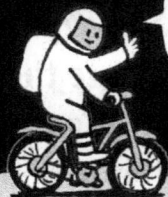

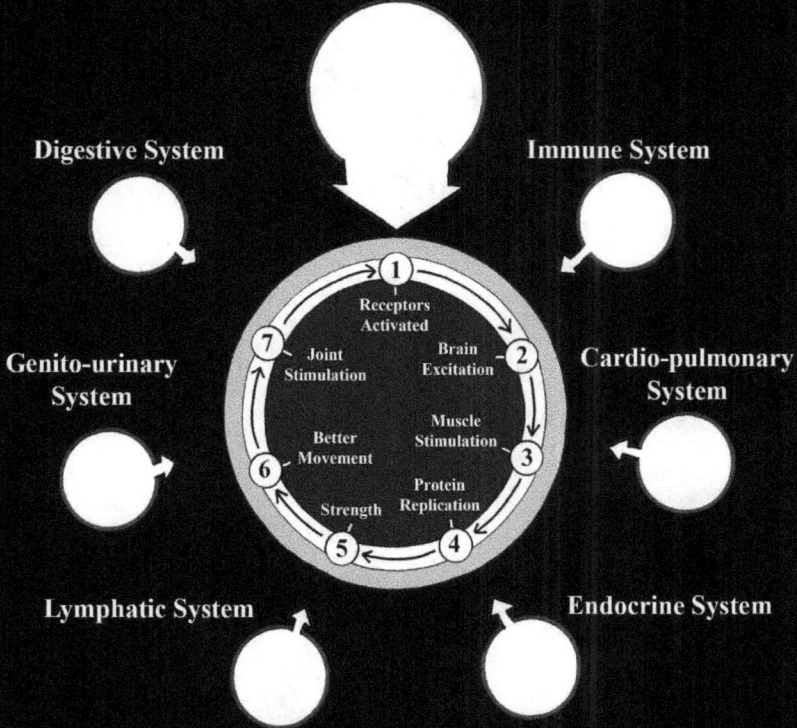

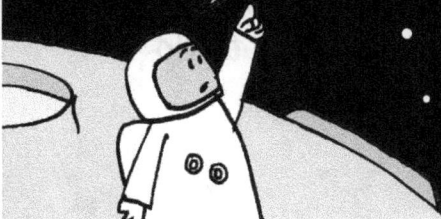

5 keys to the very best you

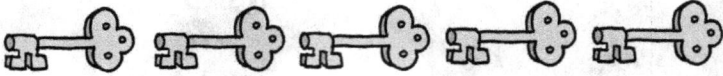

The good news is that most of these keys are already in your pocket.

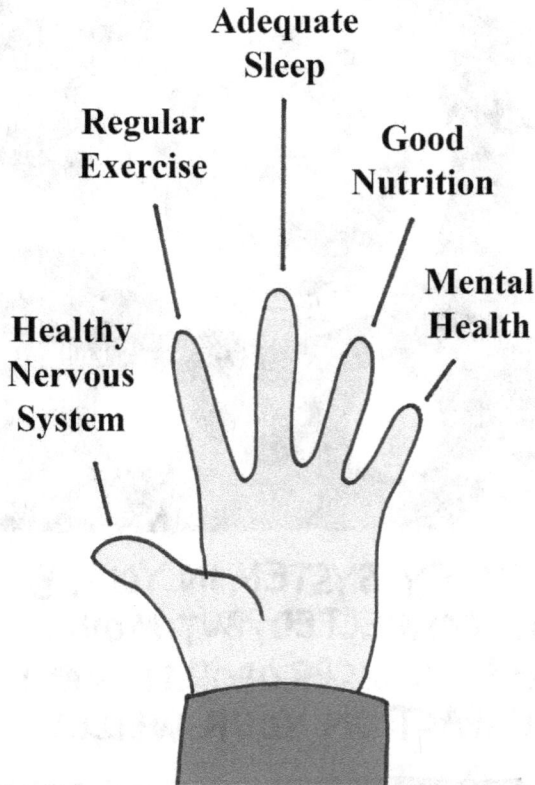

Adequate
Sleep

Regular
Exercise

Good
Nutrition

Mental
Health

Healthy
Nervous
System

From here on we will focus on easy-to-do exercises that you can do at home.

Introducing your two best friends

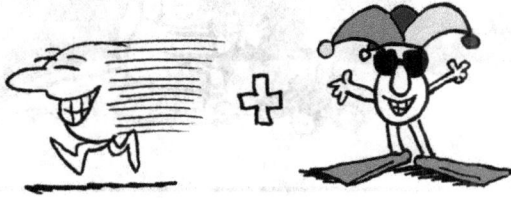

Movement and Novelty

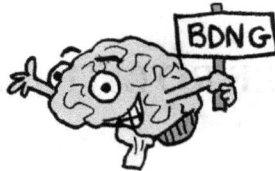

Your brain depends on them for
Brain Derived Neurotropic Growth factor
Movement creates it
Novelty preserves it

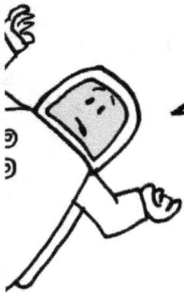

WHAT DOES THIS MEAN?

It means it's time to get moving with the following exercises.

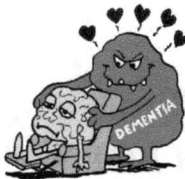

Did you know that dementia loves inactivity and boredom?

But hates movement and novelty!

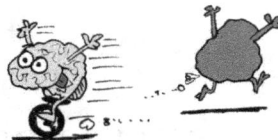

Let's get going! The choice is always yours.

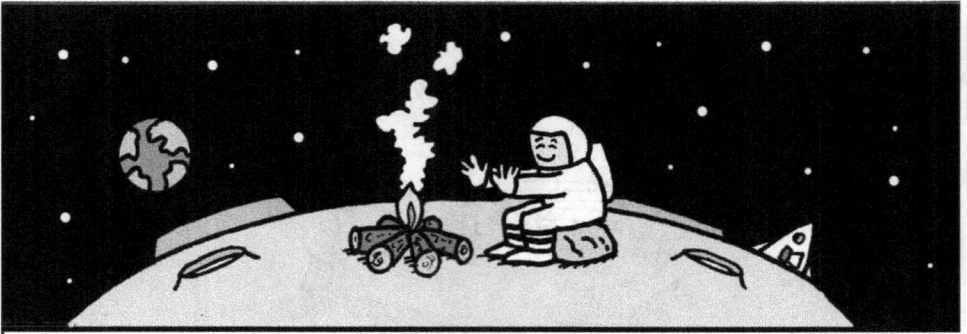

WARM UPS

1-ANKLE/KNEE ROTATIONS

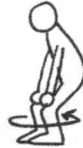

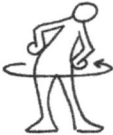

2-HIP & LOW BACK ROTATION

3-HEAD & NECK ROTATION

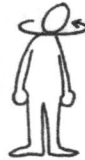

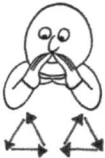

4-COMBINATION PURSUIT & VOR

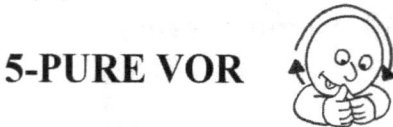

5-PURE VOR

6-VISUAL PURSUIT WITH BODY MOTION

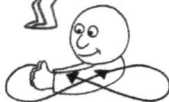

7-VISUAL PURSUIT WITH CONVERGING & DIVERGING

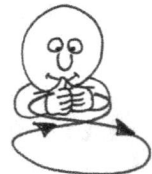

8 - CROSS CRAWLS

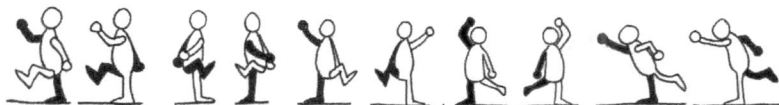

9 - ABDOMINAL HOLLOWING AND CROSS EXTENSION

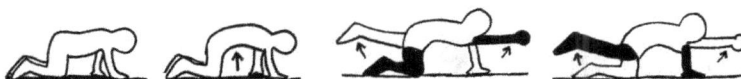

10 - MODIFIED NECK BRIDGES

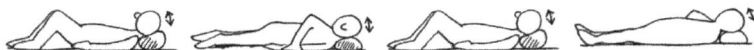

11 - FULCRUM TORQUE PROCEDURE

Requires FTP Balls

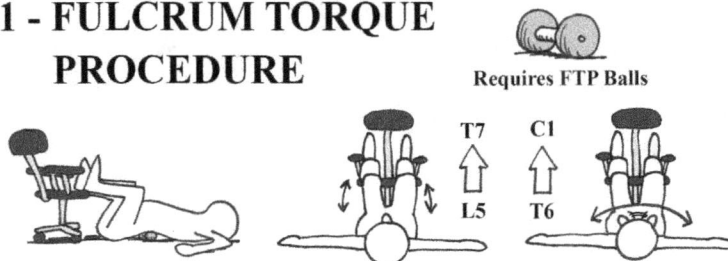

T7   C1

L5   T6

12 - SUPINE CROSS CRAWL CO-CONTRACTIONS

Left
Side
Demo

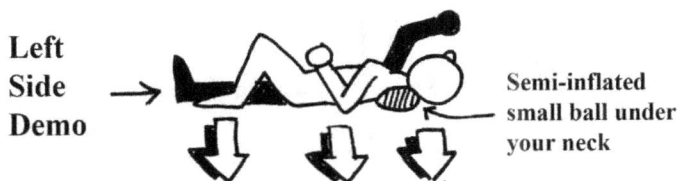

Semi-inflated
small ball under
your neck

CHEST & SHOULDERS

cs1   Incline Bench

With the band wrapped around your back and grabbing the ends in both hands extend upward at 45 degrees, exhaling as you extend and inhaling as you smoothly retract.

10 TIMES

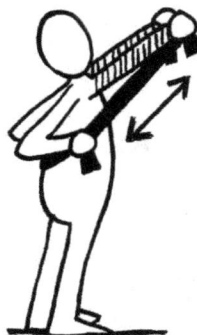

cs2   Lateral Deltoid Raise

While standing on the band with your opposite foot raise and lower your arm to the side. Do not raise your elbow higher than your shoulder to avoid stressing your shoulder. As always, exhale on the stretch, inhale on the return.

10 TIMES/EACH SIDE

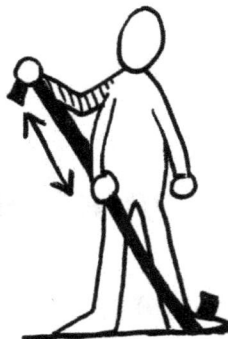

cs3   Repeat Incline Bench (cs1)

cs4   Repeat Lateral Deltoid Raise (cs2)

Throughout these exercises you will be alternating between sets of exercises in order to rest certain muscles while using others. This will add an aerobic component as well as compress the time required to complete the routines.

CHEST & SHOULDERS

cs5 Flat Bench

With the band wrapped around your back and grabbing the ends in both hands extend straight out in front of you, exhaling as you extend and inhaling as you smoothly retract.

10 TIMES

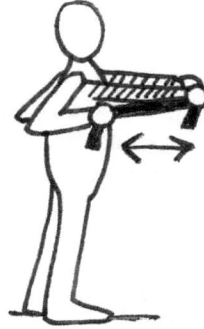

cs6 Posterior Deltoid Flys

While standing on the band with one foot raise and lower both your arms out and up.

10 TIMES

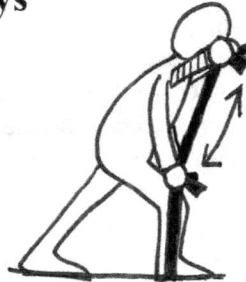

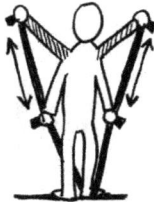

As viewed from the rear

cs7 Repeat Flat Bench (cs5)

cs7a As an advanced alternative do push-ups instead

cs8 Repeat Posterior Deltoid Flys (cs6)

CHEST & SHOULDERS

cs9 Single Arm Military Press

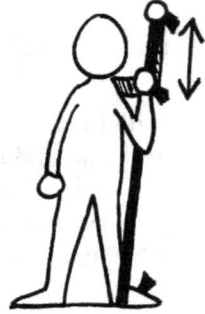

With the band under your foot and behind your arm extend up and down smoothly without raising your elbow above your shoulder.

10 TIMES/EACH ARM

cs10 Shoulder External Rotation

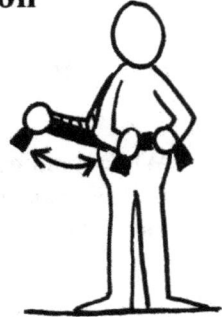

Grasp the band in both hands. With one hand rotate your arm outward, keeping your elbow close to your body. Remember to always exhale on the extention and inhale on the smooth return.

10 TIMES/EACH ARM

cs11 Repeat Single Arm Press (cs9)

cs12 Repeat Shoulder Rotation (cs10)

cs13 Shoulder Shrugs

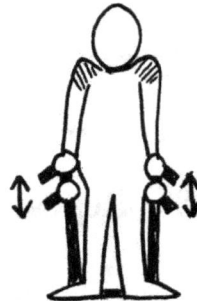

With band under both feet grasp the ends and tug up and down while keeping your arms close to your body.

10 TIMES

CHEST & SHOULDERS

cs14   Cross Crawls

As if marching in place, raise your opposite arm and leg

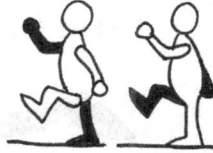

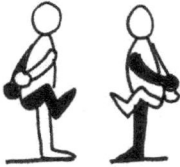

Lift your leg, crossing in front at a 45 degree angle as you cross opposite arm

Lift your leg outward at a 45 degree angle as you raise opposite arm

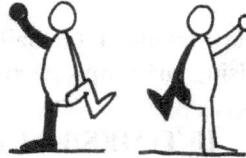

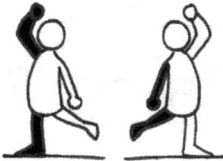

Lift your opposite arm and leg out to the side

Lift your opposite arm and leg, extending your leg straight back

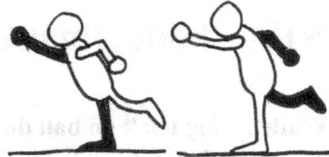

10 TIMES

cs15   Repeat Shoulder Shrugs (cs13)

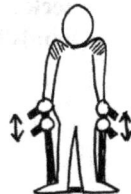

cs16   Repeat Cross Crawls (cs14)

CHEST & SHOULDERS

cs17　Abdominal Hollowing On Ball (with Cross Extention)

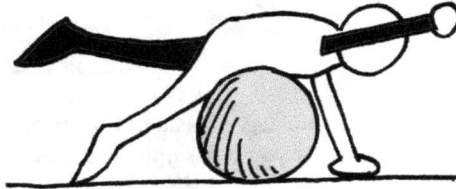

While laying on the ball alternate raising your opposite arm and leg

10 TIMES/EACH SIDE

If balancing is too difficult, do the exercise on the floor without the ball as you did in your warm ups.

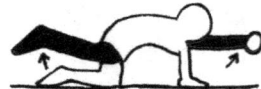

cs18　Abdominal Crunches

While laying back on ball do partial sit-ups with hands on belly. If more neck support is needed place your hands behind your head.

2 SETS OF 15

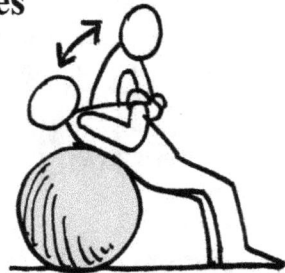

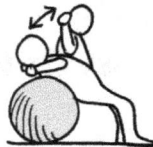

ARMS & BACK

ab1   Single Arm Bicep Curl

While standing on band pull up in a curl position. Remember to exhale during the stretch and inhale while smoothly lowering your arm.

10 TIMES/EACH SIDE

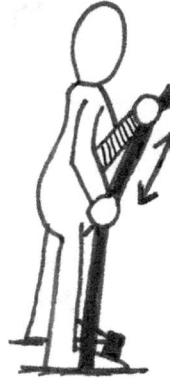

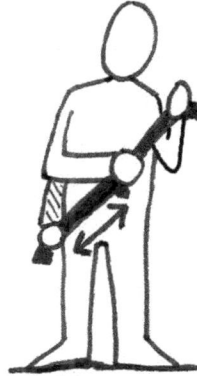

ab2   Single Arm Tricep Extension

While holding the band in your opposite hand at shoulder height grab it with your other hand mid-chest. From there pull down to your side and back.

10 TIMES/EACH SIDE

ab3   Repeat Single Arm Curl (ab1)

ab4   Repeat Tricep Extension (ab2)

ARMS & BACK

ab5   Wrist Extension

While kneeling with one arm on
your leg wrap the band around your
hand in a fist, palm down. With the
other hand hold tension as you pivot
up and down.

10 TIMES/EACH SIDE

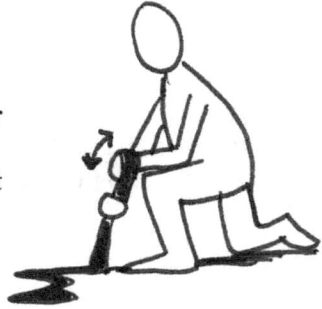

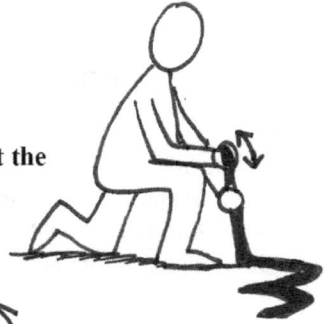

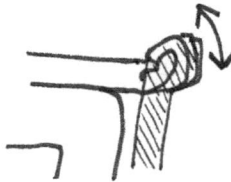

ab6   Wrist Flexion

While in the same position rotate your
wrist to the upright position and repeat the
previous exercise.

10 TIMES/EACH SIDE

ab7   Repeat Wrist Extension (ab5)

ab8   Repeat Wrist Flexion (ab6)

ARMS & BACK

ab9   Finger Extention With Abduction

Continuing with the same posture
wrap the band around your splayed
out fingers and repeat the process,
palm down.

10 TIMES/EACH SIDE

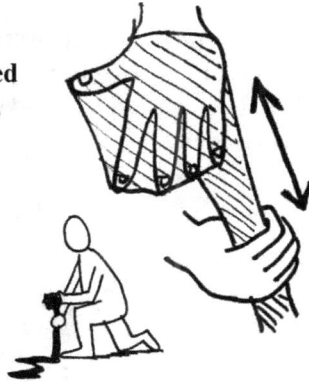

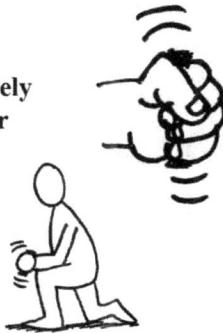

ab10   Finger Flexion

The last kneeling exercise involved merely
wadding up the band tightly inside your
fist and squeezing.

10 TIMES/EACH SIDE

ab11   Repeat Finger Extension (ab9)

ab12   Repeat FingerFlexion (ab10)

ARMS & BACK

ab13   Lat Press On Ball

Cradling the large ball under your
arm, steadying with your opposite
hand. Then push down into the ball
with your elbow.

10 TIMES/EACH SIDE

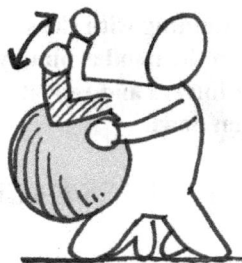

ab14   Dead Lifts

Starting from a squat, standing on the
band with legs apart, grab both ends and
stand straight up. Repeat ten times.

10 TIMES

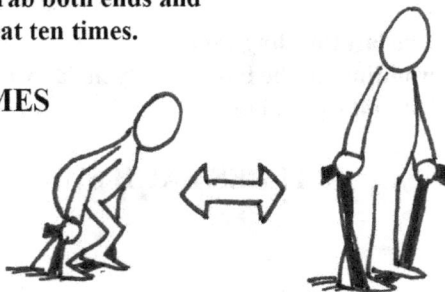

ab15   Repeat Lat Press On Ball (ab13)

ab16   Repeat Dead Lifts (ab14)

ARMS & BACK

ab17   Seated Row

Sitting on the floor wrap the band
around the bottom of your feet.
Once your legs are extended sit
upright and pull back and forth as if
rowing.

10 TIMES

For a greater challenge try doing it
while sitting on the ball.

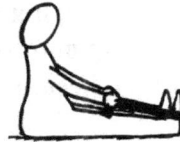

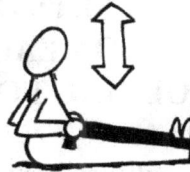

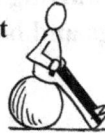

ab18   Reverse Lunges

Starting from a standing position lunge
backwards to the height of a seated
position and back up again.

10 TIMES/EACH LEG

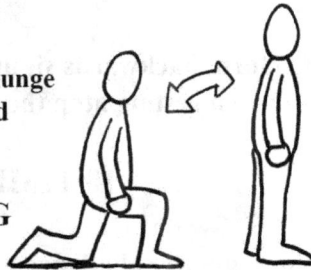

ab19   Repeat Seated Row (ab17)

ab20   Repeat Reverse Lunges (ab18)

ARMS & BACK

ab21   Side Plank

From a side lying position hoist yourself up onto your forearm and your toes, keeping your body rigid.

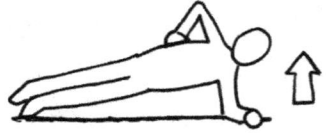

2 SETS OF 5 REPS
ON EACH SIDE
HOLDING FOR 8 SECONDS

If too difficult try starting out doing them with your legs and hip still on the floor.

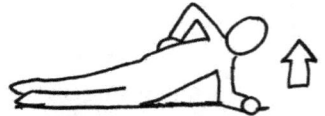

ab22   Extension Low Back On Ball

Perform backwards sit ups with your stomach resting atop the ball.

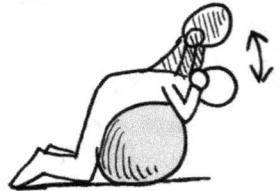

10 TIMES

For a greater challenge extend your legs until you are on your toes.

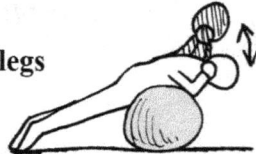

ab23   Repeat Side Plank (ab21)

ab24   Repeat Extension On Ball (ab22)

LEGS

lg1 Squats With Bands

With the band under one foot descend into a mock seated position and straighten up again. Remember to eshale on the stretch and inhale on the descent.

10-12 TIMES

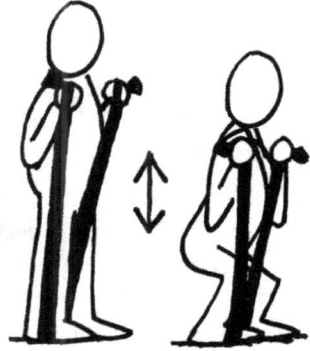

lg2 Ankle Alphabet

LIft one leg just off the ground and, by wiggling your foot, spell the alphabet in its entirety: upper case, lower case or cursive. It's your choice.

A to Z WITH EACH FOOT

To aid in balance you can hold onto a chair if necessary.

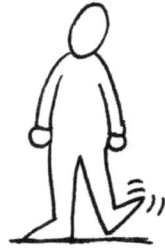

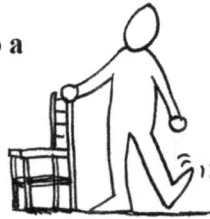

lg3 Repeat Squats With Bands (lg1)

lg4 Repeat Ankle Alphabet (lg2)

LEGS

lg5 Calf & Anterior Leg Combination

Start by tying the ends of your band together and then twisting it into a figure 8. Then sit on the floor and wrap the band around both feet. Alternate one leg up and down as you take turns alternating reps: Lower foot - toe pushing away. Upper foot toe - pulling toward you.

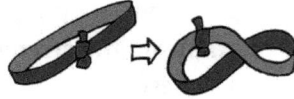

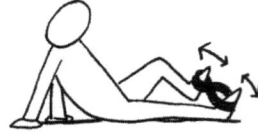

**10 TIMES EACH
THEN SWITCH LEGS**

Both legs up for advanced workout.

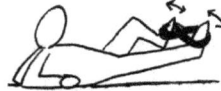

lg6 Ankle Eversion/Inversion

Twist ankle outward, one foot at a time.

10 TIME EACH FOOT

Then cross one leg over the other and take turns twisting each ankle inwardly.

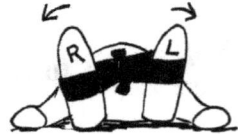

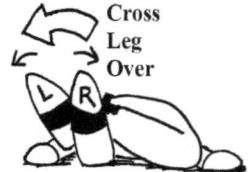

lg7 Repeat Calf /Ant. Leg Combo (lg5)

lg8 Repeat Ankle Eversion/Inversion (lg6)

LEGS

lg9   Abductor-Squeeze Ball

With the ball between your legs
squeeze inwardly. Remember to
exhale on the squeeze and inhales as
you relax.

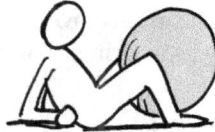

10-12 TIMES

Airborne ball is optional.

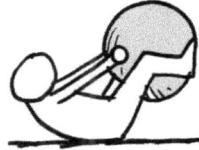

lg10   Hamstring Supine Legs On Ball

With your legs on top of the ball press your
heels into the ball. Hold the pressure for
about one second each time.

10-12 TIMES

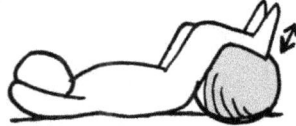

lg11   Repeat Abductor-Squeeze Ball (lg9)

lg12   Repeat Hamstring Legs On Ball (lg10)

LEGS

lg13   Ab Hollowing On Ball With
Cross Extension

While arched over ball alternate
left-right arm and leg extensions

**5 TIMES EACH SIDE
FOR A TOTAL OF 10
EXTENSIONS**

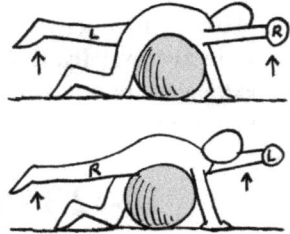

lg14   Abdominal - Kneel In Front Of Ball

Kneeling in front of the ball, lean over it
and press your elbows into it. exhaling on
the press and inhaling as you relax.

10 TIMES

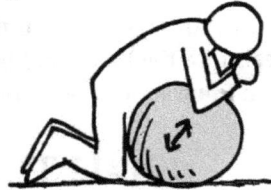

lg15   Repeat Hollowing On Ball (lg13)

lg16   Repeat Abdominal -Front of Ball (lg14)

SPECIAL PROCEDURE

Passive Neck Extension

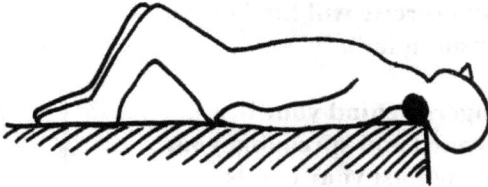

Lie down on your back with cylindrical support under your neck. Relax as you allow your neck to stretch backwards off the end of your bed.

2,4,6...ULTIMATELY 20 MINUTES/DAILY

Start with several minutes and gradually increase the duration each time you do it. It requires 15 to 18 minutes to stretch out the front of your cervical vertebra. The benefits of restoring the natural curvature in your neck will prove more than worth it.

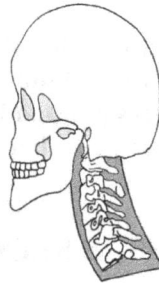

BEWARE OF TEXTING NECK

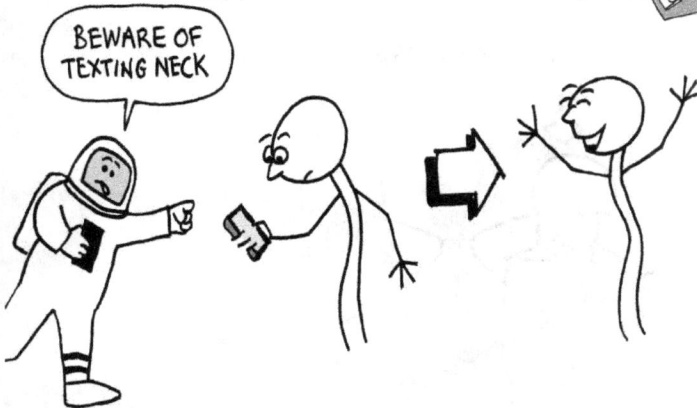

LAST BUT NOT LEAST

Resistant Neck Extension A

While sitting or standing throughout the day this 30 second exercise will further help you to avoid the "slumpies".

Interlace your fingers behind your head. While looking upward and spreading your elbows press back against your hands.

3 TIMES - 5 SECONDS EACH

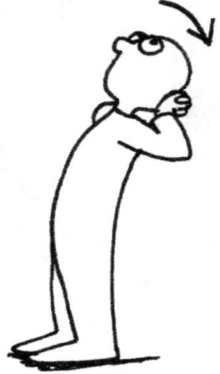

Resistant Neck Extention B

Then shift your hands to a prayerful position, still behind your head, with your fingers pointed backwards. Once again press back against your hands.

2 TIMES - 5 SECONDS EACH

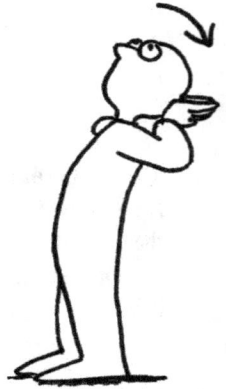

REAR VIEWS

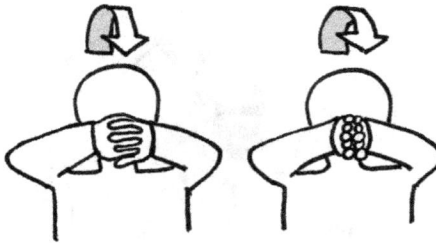

A   B

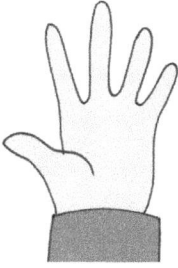

IT'S IN YOUR HANDS

Remember the five keys to the very best you. Together they form a force field that will protect your health and wellbeing.

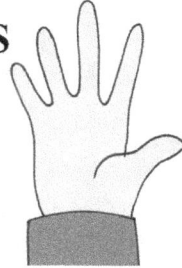

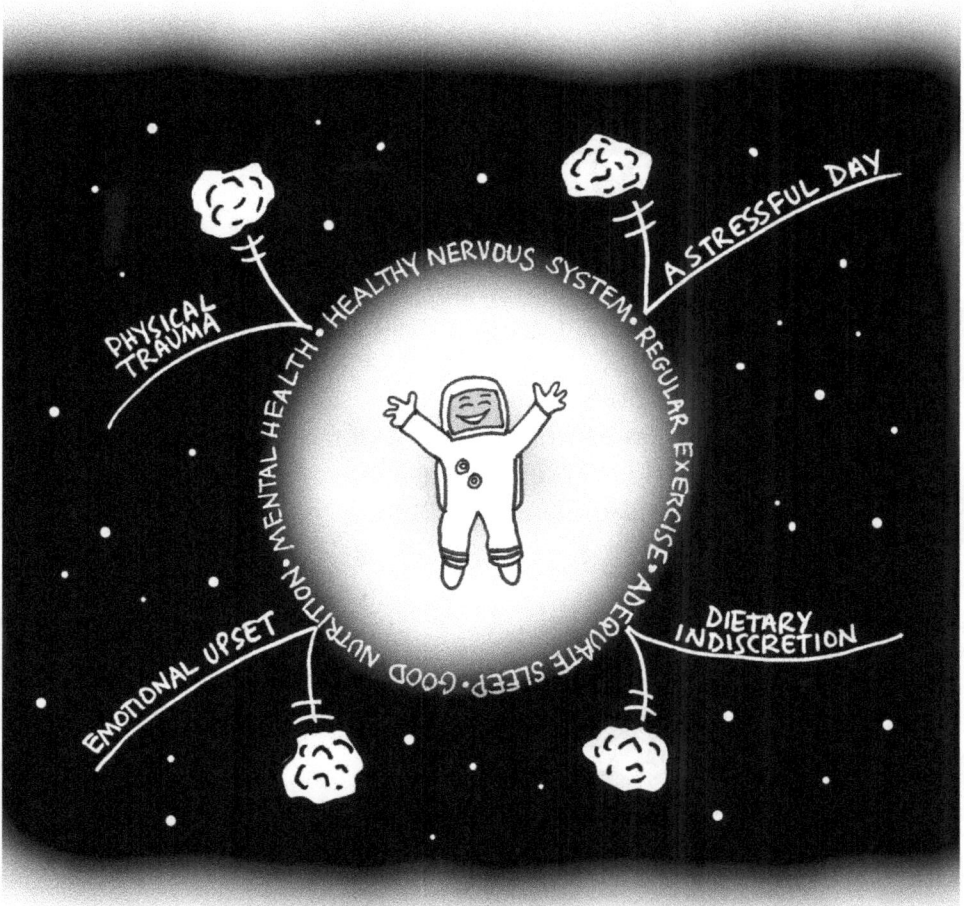

Stay strong and live well!

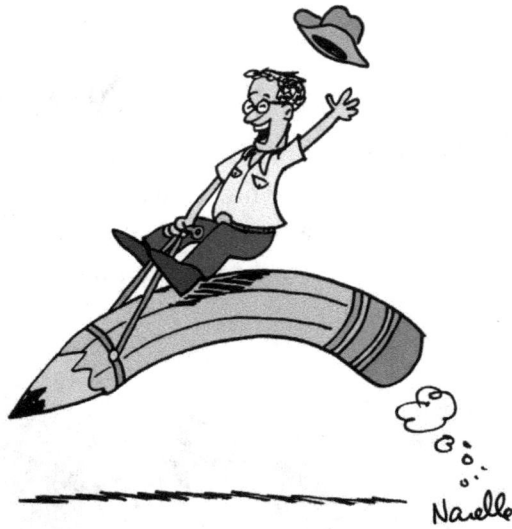

Brian Narelle began cartooning at the age of eight. No one ever told him to stop, so he didn't. He specializes in making complicated things digestible, be it IBM technology or emergency medicine, and has illustrated many books. As a writer he started out on Sesame Street and has gone on to write award winning PBS Specials and dozens of educational film. Coming full circle, he currently teaches cartooning to eight-year-olds at the Charles Schulz Museum in California.

Brian Narelle
briannarelle@comcast.net
Narellecreative.com
707.586.2070

Visit THENEUROTECHNOLOGIES.COM
for more resources

Check out Book 1 and Book 2 in the
Brain Back Body Series!
Also available in Spanish

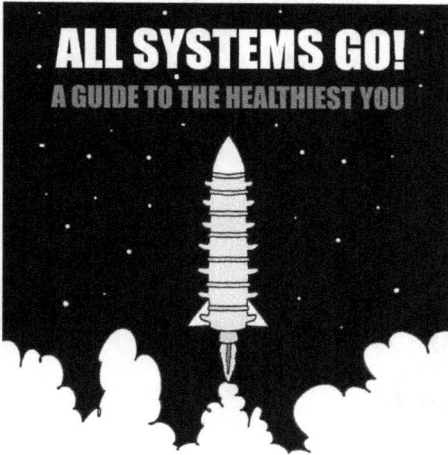

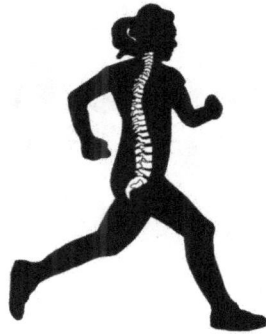

www.ingramcontent.com/pod-product-compliance
Lightning Source LLC
Chambersburg PA
CBHW060531280326
41933CB00014B/3136